Mindfulness for Kids I

7 Children's Meditations & Mindfulness Practices to Help Kids Be More Focused, Calm and Relaxed

Dr. Nicola Kluge, Ph.D.

The Arts & Education Foundation, Houston, Texas

Published by the Arts and Education Foundation, Houston, Texas

ISBN-10: 0991212711
ISBN-13: 978-0991212712

For Free Mindfulness Activities
Connect with Us at
MindfulnessForKids.net

Check out our "Mindfulness For Kids" series: books, CDs and MP3s.

If you enjoyed this book please leave a review online.
Thank you for your support!

Dedication

This book is dedicated to my parents Eva & Karl,
to my children Mattan, Noa, Marko & Milan,
and to my husband Jack, who is an Angel walking this earth.
Thank you for your love and support!

Contents

Note to Parents and Teachers

In this chapter, I will briefly explain how Mindfulness Meditation is helpful to children. I will talk about what to expect during the meditation process, and how to use your voice reading the meditation story. I will also introduce you to optional Warm-up and Follow-up activities that can help deepen the benefits of meditation.

What Is Mindfulness

Mindfulness is noticing what comes through our senses during any activity; for example, sounds in our environment, breathing, or looking at something and noticing details (i.e. size, colors, and textures), etc. Distracting thoughts and feelings are not ignored but rather acknowledged and observed without judgment.

Why Teach Mindfulness to Children

Mindfulness Meditation can have many benefits. Research has shown that meditating can help children:

- Feel peaceful & tranquil
- Fall asleep more easily
- Cope with stress & anxiety
- Increase focus & concentration
- Improve relationships
- Handle difficult emotions
- Develop creativity & imagination
- Learn to quiet themselves

When you practice Mindfulness Meditation together with children, you will better understand their perspective and needs and, as an added benefit, become closer in your relationship.

About the Mindfulness Meditation Process

Please see the Warm-up activities, Mindfulness Meditations, discussion questions, and Creative Arts projects enclosed in this book as ideas for your own Mindfulness practice with your child or the students in your class. They are meant for you to incorporate them into your classroom routine or your practice at home.

The ideas in this book are not meant to represent a complete Mindfulness Meditation session from beginning to end, but can be a helpful addition to your own routine or can serve as an introduction to Mindfulness. Please feel free to modify the activities to suit your needs.

Each story in the "Mindfulness for Kids" series contains a visualization of a light source to focus children's attention and start the relaxation process. This source of light can be the moon, a star, the sun, a campfire, etc.

Children are encouraged to visualize and feel the warm light throughout their body, relax their muscles, and quiet their thoughts. Children are invited to experience loving thoughts towards themselves and others.

In many of the meditation stories in this book, children are welcomed by their own unique Guide or friend. This can be an older wise person, a Guardian Angel, an animal, or an imaginary being. Each child can decide who or what their Guide or friend is. The Guide or friend is there to help children feel safe and protected.

As a parent, when you do a meditation in the evening or at night, leave your child at a place in the story where they can drift into sleep.

During the day or when in the classroom, continue reading the story to the end. Have children become fully alert and present, and then continue with your daily routine.

How to Use Your Voice

Please read the meditation scripts slowly and with a relaxed, soothing tone of voice. Pause frequently (I indicate where in the book), and let children experience the scene you just set. Give children plenty of time to experience what they see, hear, and feel.

Warm-up & Follow-up Activities

In this book you will find fun Warm-up activities to prepare children for the meditation process and the meditation story. You will also find activities to help children process thoughts and feelings after the meditation.

All suggested activities are optional. However, they can significantly help children understand their experience as well as deepen the effects and benefits of meditation.

When you ask the suggested questions, react to children's answers in an understanding, non-judgmental way. These are open-ended, explorative questions. There are no wrong answers.

Also, let children choose their meditation posture. Children can lie down, sit, kneel, keep their eyes open or closed, etc. as long as they are comfortable.

Thank you for sharing the benefits of Mindfulness with children!

Children's Mindfulness Meditation 1: Water Lily - Gentle Relaxation

Ages: 5-12 ~ Meditation: 5-10 min. ~ Activities: 30-45 min.

Warm-up, Meditation & Follow-up Activities

I. Warm-up

Introduction of Topic:

- Bring pictures or books about water lilies. Talk about what you see on the pictures. Talk about color, shape, size, etc.
- Talk about the different plant parts (i.e. blossoms, stems, roots, etc.) and their importance.

Opening questions:

To spike interest in the upcoming meditation, ask questions like:

- Can you remember a time when you floated in water? Please share! What does it feel like?
- Do you like cold water or warm water?
- What does a water lily need to grow?
- How come a water lily can float in the water without floating away?
- How does a flower blossom open? Show with your hands!
- If you were a water lily what color would you be? What would you smell like? Who would your friends be?

Give children time to think and answer each question!

Fun Activities:

Please choose one of the following activities:

- Give children small trinkets and things that float. Prepare a small tub filled with water. Have children experiment with things that float in the tub. Show them how to make gentle waves in the water.
- Have children experience tension and relaxation. Ask them to make fists with both hands, hold them for several seconds, and then let go and relax. Again, make fists, hold them, and then let go. What does it feel like?

II. Mindfulness Meditation 1: Water Lily - Gentle Relaxation

- Encourage (but don't force!) children to close or cover their eyes during the meditation.
- Have children choose their own meditation posture (i.e. sitting, laying, etc.). Let them choose a meditation position they feel most comfortable with.
- Turn to page 11 for the meditation script. Read thoughtfully; allow time for children to process what they are experiencing while you are reading.
- When you are done reading, give children time to slowly "wake up" and stretch. When all children are fully alert, continue with the Follow-up activities outlined below.

III. Follow-up Activities

Discussion Questions:

Discussing what children experienced during meditation can help with processing thoughts and feelings, thus deepening the effects.

Here are ideas for conversation topics:

- How are you feeling?
- What was your favorite part of the story?
- What color was your water lily? How big was it, etc.?
- Would you want to be a water lily for a little while? Why?
- What did you experience during the meditation (i.e. see, hear, feel)?
- How will you use what you experienced in this meditation in your daily life? Concretely, when, where, and how will you use it?

Please remember: there are no wrong answers. Simply thank children for contributing to the question or ask them to describe the experience further.

Creative Arts Projects:

Creative Arts Projects can deepen the effects and understanding of children's meditation. The following are ideas to do together.

Please choose one of the following activities:

- Draw or paint a water lily or water lilies floating on top of a pond.
- Draw or paint a flower awakened by sunshine.
- Make a flower out of tissue paper or crêpe paper. Use pipe cleaners or other art supplies as stems.
- Draw or paint a picture of the experiences or feelings you had during the meditation.
- Pretend you are a water lily sleeping – how do you wake up when the sun rises and gently awakens you?

Encourage children to share their project with the group!

Meditation Script 1: Water Lily - Gentle Relaxation

Imagine you are a water lily floating peacefully on top of a pond's gentle waters. (Pause)
The water feels warm from the rays of the sun.
You feel very relaxed and comfortable. (Pause)

Notice the fragrance of the water lilies around you.
They are your friends. (Pause)

Notice how light your body feels. (Pause)

At the same time, notice how strong your roots are.
Feel how firmly they are connected to the ground at the bottom of the pond.
These roots help you feel safe and secure. (Pause)

Take in the warm rays of the sun.
Imagine your petals slowly open one by one. (Pause)

Take all the time you need to open your flower. (Pause)
With each petal that opens, warm golden sunlight floods in and fills your heart with love and joy. (Pause)
Feel how the sun's light and warmth expand throughout all your body. (Pause)

Take a moment and feel the golden light travel and expand:
from your head, (Pause)
to your arms, (Pause)
to your feet, (Pause)
and your toes. (Pause)
Take a deep breath in, and fully open your heart to the sun.
Notice how peaceful you feel. (Pause)

As you breathe out, send:
peace, (Pause)
love, (Pause)
and light (Pause)
from your heart to the people around you, (Pause)
and to someone who you know needs extra love today. (Pause)

Take a moment to notice how you feel. (Pause)
Know that you can always come back to this place. (Pause)

If your eyes are closed, open them whenever you are ready.
Feeling fully alert, yet very relaxed.

Children's Mindfulness Meditation 2:
Music to My Ears – Sound Mindfulness Practice

Ages: 5-12 ~ Meditation: 5-10 min. ~ Activities: 30-45 min.

Warm-up, Meditation & Follow-up Activities

I. Warm-up

Introduction of Topic:

Please choose one of the following activities:

- Bring in a Tibetan Bell or Singing Bowl. Have children take turns touching and experimenting with it. Discuss the experience.
- Bring various small musical instruments, such as egg shakers, small bells, and tambourines. Have children take turns touching and experimenting with the instruments. Discuss the experience.
- Play short excerpts of music from different genres. Discuss how each piece makes the children feel and what their thoughts are.

Opening questions:

To spike interest in the upcoming meditation, ask questions like:

- How do we hear?
- Can you feel sound?
- How can different sounds make you feel? Have children come up with examples.

Give children time to think and answer each question!

Fun Activities:

Please choose one of the following activities:

- Have children listen to a Tibetan Bell or Singing Bowl. Discuss the experience.
- Have children close their eyes and listen to different sounds they hear inside and outside the room. Talk about what they heard.
- Bring in things that make different sounds, but don't show the children. Have them close their eyes and listen to each sound you make. Have them guess what it is. Discuss the experience.
- Practice the "Om" sound with the children. Become aware of the sensations your body experiences when producing the sound. Discuss the experience.

II. Mindfulness Meditation 2: Music to My Ears – Sound Mindfulness Practice

Preparation: Prepare a 10-15 minute piece of calming music - classical music works great for this. Make sure you listen to the music you pick before playing music that is unsuitable for children.

- Encourage (but don't force!) children to close or cover their eyes during the meditation.
- Have children choose their own meditation posture (i.e. sitting, laying, etc.). Let them choose a meditation position they feel most comfortable with.
- Turn to page 14 for the meditation script. Read thoughtfully; allow time for children to process what they are experiencing while you are reading.
- When you are done reading, give children time to slowly "wake up" and stretch. When all children are fully alert, continue with the Follow-up activities outlined below.

III. Follow-up Activities

Discussion Questions:

Discussing what children experienced during meditation can help with processing thoughts and feelings, thus deepening the effects.

Here are ideas for conversation topics:

- How are you feeling?
- What did you experience during the meditation (i.e. see, hear, feel)?
- How will you use what you experienced in this meditation in your daily life? Concretely, when, where, and how will you use it?

Please remember: there are no wrong answers. Simply thank children for contributing to the question or ask them to describe the experience further.

Creative Arts Projects:

Creative Arts Projects can deepen the effects and understanding of children's meditation. The following are ideas to do together.

Please choose one of the following activities:

- Draw, paint, or make a collage out of magazine clippings of the sounds or music you heard and experienced.
- Draw, paint, or make a collage out of magazine clippings of what the music tasted like, smelled like, or looked like.
- Draw, paint, or make a collage out of magazine clippings of the experiences or feelings you had during the meditation.

Encourage children to share their projects with the group!

Meditation Script 2: Music to My Ears – Sound Mindfulness Practice

Begin by focusing your attention on your breath.
Notice the air when you breathe in and out. (Pause)

Feel you tummy rise when you breathe in.
Feel your tummy relax when you breathe out. (Pause)

Breathe in and out. (Pause)

Relax your muscles.
Feel them become soft and relaxed with every breath you take. (Pause)
Breathe in and out. (Pause)

Now, bring your awareness to what you are hearing.
Notice the music or the sounds inside and outside your room. (Pause)

How do you experience them?
Pleasant? Unpleasant? Or neutral? (Pause)

Now, tune in to the music you hear. (Pause)
How does the music make you feel?
Comfortable? Uncomfortable? (Pause)

Notice how the music touches your ears.
Do you hear high notes? Or low notes? (Pause)

Do you feel like you want the music to be louder?
Or do you want it softer? (Pause)

Does the music you hear remind you of anyone or anything?
A place? An event? (Pause)

What thoughts do you notice while listening to the music? (Pause)
Say *Hello*! to your thoughts.
Then, let them go and see them drift away with the sound of the music. (Pause)

How does your body react to the music? (Pause)
How does your tummy feel?
How about your heart beat?
What is your body telling you? (Pause)

Now, join me for a fun experiment:

Imagine feeling the music with your nose!
Breathe the music in.
Breathe the music out.
Smell the music.
What does it smell like? (Pause)

Now, see the music with your eyes.
See the music in beautiful colors and images.
What colors do you see?
What images come to mind? (Pause)

Now, feel the music with your mouth.
What does the music taste like?
How does it feel on your tongue?
Does it taste like something you like? (Pause)

Take all the time you need to hear, (Pause)
see, (Pause)
smell, (Pause)
taste, (Pause)
and feel the music. (Pause)

Thank your body for allowing you to experience the world, and yourself, through your senses.
Thank your body for taking care of you. (Pause)

If your eyes are closed, open them whenever you are ready.
Feeling fully alert, yet very relaxed.

Children's Mindfulness Meditation 3: Power Shield – Loving Kindness Practice

Ages: 6-12 ~ Meditation: 5-10 min. ~ Activities: 30-45 min.

Warm-up, Meditation & Follow-up Activities

I. Warm-up

Opening questions:

To spike interest in the upcoming meditation, ask questions like:

- What are your three most favorite feelings, and why?
- What is Loving Kindness? What does it feel like?
- What are examples of loving, caring thoughts or acts towards others or yourself?
- How can Loving Kindness make you strong inside and out?

Give children time to think and answer each question!

Fun Activity:
- Have children come up with examples of acts of Loving Kindness.
- Read a book, newspaper, magazine article, or show children pictures of someone doing something kind to someone else. Discuss what you read or observed.

II. Mindfulness Meditation 3: Power Shield – Loving Kindness Practice

- Encourage (but don't force!) children to close or cover their eyes during the meditation.
- Have children choose their own meditation posture (i.e. sitting, laying, etc.). Let them choose a meditation position they feel most comfortable with.
- Turn to page 18 for the meditation script. Read thoughtfully; allow time for children to process what they are experiencing while you are reading.
- When you are done reading, give children time to slowly "wake up" and stretch. When all children are fully alert, continue with the Follow-up activities outlined below.

III. Follow-up Activities

Discussion Questions:

Discussing what children experienced during meditation can help with processing thoughts and feelings, thus deepening the effects.

Here are ideas for conversation topics:

- How are you feeling?
- What did you experience during the meditation (i.e. see, hear, feel)?
- How will you use what you experienced in this meditation in your daily life? Concretely, when, where, and how will you use it?

Additional questions you might ask:

- What did your Power Shield look like?
- What did your Power Shield feel like?
- Who would you share your Power Shield with? Why?
- What else would you like your Power Shield to do for you?

Please remember: there are no wrong answers. Simply thank children for contributing to the question or ask them to describe the experience further.

Creative Arts Projects:

Creative Arts Projects can deepen the effects and understanding of children's meditation. The following are ideas to do together.

Please choose one of the following activities:

- Draw, paint, or make a collage out of magazine clippings of your Power Shield.
- Make a Power Shield out of heavy card stock, construction paper, or cardboard. Decorate it.
- Draw, paint, or make a collage out of magazine clippings of the experiences or feelings you had during the meditation.
- Create a command (i.e. snapping fingers, whistling, clapping, or saying a word) for your Power Shield to appear whenever you want it to.

Encourage children to share their projects with the group!

Meditation Script 3: Power Shield – Loving Kindness Practice

Gently place one hand on your tummy. (Pause)

Feel your tummy rise when you breathe in.
Relax as you breathe out. (Pause)

Again, breathe in and feel your tummy rise.
Breathe out, feel your tummy relax. (Pause)

One more time: Breathe in, feel your tummy rise.
Breathe out, relax. (Pause)

Now, imagine a tiny, warm, golden light around your tummy area where you placed your hand. (Pause)

With every breath you take, see the tiny warm golden light grow bigger and bigger,
until you see yourself immersed in it:
from head to toe, (Pause)
and all around you. (Pause)

Feel this radiant, golden, loving light shine from within you. (Pause)

This is your Power Shield. (Pause)

Make your Power Shield even stronger by adding your favorite feelings to it. (Pause)
See, hear, and feel your favorite feelings become part of the Power Shield around you and the loving light
within you. (Pause)

Now, hear, see, and feel things that make you feel good about yourself. (Pause)
Notice your Power Shield and the loving light within you become even bigger and stronger. (Pause)

Now, see, hear, and feel your favorite wishes.
These are wishes that are loving and caring towards yourself, other people, animals, plants, and
the Universe. (Pause)
Notice the Power Shield and the loving light within you grow even bigger and stronger. (Pause)

Take a deep breath in. Feel your tummy rise. See the light glow brighter.
Breathe out. Feel your tummy relax.
See the light swirl all around you. (Pause)

Now, place your hand on your heart. (Pause)

Imagine hearing yourself say: With this light that is always with me -
"May I be safe.
May I be happy.
May I be healthy.
May I be peaceful."

Take a moment and notice how you feel. (Pause)

May the love and peacefulness you experienced be with you, always, and in all ways. (Pause)

If your eyes are closed, open them whenever you are ready.
Feeling fully alert, yet very relaxed.

Children's Mindfulness Meditation 4: Star Child – Calm Focus

Ages: 5-12 ~ Meditation: 10-15 min. ~ Activities: 30-45 min.

Warm-up, Meditation & Follow-up Activities

I. Warm-up

Opening questions:

To spike interest in the upcoming meditation, ask questions like:

- What is your favorite color?
- How does color influence us or impact our lives? (i.e. traffic light: red means stop; green means go; yellow means alert) What other examples can you come up with?
- What does the color red (or green, orange, brown, etc.) mean to you?
- When I say the color "blue" (or red, purple, green, etc.) what is the first thing you think of?
- What is a happy (or quiet, refreshing, angry, etc.) color?

Give children time to think and answer each question!

Fun Activity:

- Have children play and experiment with a multicolored Play-Parachute. Spread the parachute out on the floor. Have children sit on their favorite color. Have another adult or child help you turn the parachute in a circle. Change direction every once in a while.

II. Mindfulness Meditation 4: Star Child – Calm Focus

- Encourage (but don't force!) children to close or cover their eyes during the meditation.
- Have children choose their own meditation posture (i.e. sitting, laying, etc.). Let them choose a meditation position they feel most comfortable with.
- Turn to page 22 for the meditation script. Read thoughtfully; allow time for children to process what they are experiencing while you are reading.
- When you are done reading, give children time to slowly "wake up" and stretch. When all children are fully alert, continue with the Follow-up activities outlined below.

III. Follow-up Activities

Discussion Questions:

Discussing what children experienced during meditation can help with processing thoughts and feelings, thus deepening the effects.

Here are ideas for conversation topics:

- How are you feeling?
- What did you experience during the meditation (i.e. see, hear, feel)?
- How will you use what you experienced in this meditation in your daily life? Concretely, when, where, and how will you use it?

Additional questions you might ask:

- Would you like to be a Star Child? What would you do?
- How would you send loving energy back to the Star Child, your grandma, your friends, etc.?

Please remember: there are no wrong answers. Simply thank children for contributing to the question or ask them to describe the experience further.

Creative Arts Projects:

Creative Arts Projects can deepen the effects and understanding of children's meditation. The following are ideas to do together.

Please choose one of the following activities:

- Make planets out of Styrofoam balls from a craft store. Paint them in your favorite color and decorate them.
- Paint a picture in your favorite color.
- Draw or paint the colors you experienced during the meditation and how they made you feel.
- Draw or paint a picture of the warm, colorful energy you experienced within and around you during the meditation.
- Draw or paint a picture of the Star Child.
- Draw or paint a picture of the planet where the Star Child lives.
- Draw or paint how you fly with the Star Child through the night sky.
- Draw or paint a picture of the experiences or feelings you had during the meditation.
- Write or draw a Thank-you letter to the Star Child.

Encourage children to share their projects with the group!

Meditation Script 4: Star Child – Calm Focus

Imagine a starry night. (Pause)
Thousands of little stars sparkle above you. (Pause)
Everything feels peaceful and quiet. (Pause)

The moon shines its silvery golden light on the trees and flowers in your imaginary garden. (Pause)

Between the branches of the old oak tree you see someone special hiding.
Can you tell who it is? (Pause)

You move closer and hear a soft giggle like the twinkle of silver bells.
Look between the leaves and see the Star Child. (Pause)

The Star Child smiles at you and waves for you to come closer. (Pause)

A gentle breeze rustles the leaves of the old oak tree as the Star Child takes you by the hand and lifts you up. (Pause)

The two of you fly to the sky to where the Star Child lives. (Pause)

Breathe in the fresh, clean night air. Relax your legs as you breathe out. (Pause)
Breathe in as you fly higher and higher. Breathe out as you relax your arms. (Pause)

See the earth getting smaller and smaller as you glide farther and farther away into the sky. (Pause)

The star where your friend the Star Child lives is made out of colorful, warm energy. (Pause)
This energy feels like some of your favorite feelings: love, joy, and peace.

Allow this colorful, warm energy to gently surround you. (Pause)

See and feel yourself immersed in all the colors. (Pause)

Notice how each of the colors makes you feel:
Red helps you feel strong and confident.
Orange makes you feel happy and excited.
Yellow helps you think and understand.
Green lets you love other people and yourself.
Blue helps you express yourself to other people.
Purple allows you to see pictures in your mind with your eyes closed.
White helps you feel included. (Pause)

Take a deep breath in and relax as you breathe out. (Pause)

See and feel yourself immersed in all the colors. (Pause)

Imagine hearing beautiful music with each color. (Pause)

Feel warm, loving energy all around you and within you. (Pause)

Know that you are loved and cared for, always. (Pause)

Know that you can always come back to this special place and continue your journey. (Pause)

As the Star Child takes you by the hand, you feel it's time to come back to your garden.
The two of you fly through the night sky and land back by the old oak tree. (Pause)

Thank the Star Child and yourself for the wonderful experience. (Pause)

Enjoy how your heart is filled with love for all beings: people, animals, plants and, of course, yourself. (Pause)

Send some of this loving energy back to the universe for the highest and greatest good. (Pause)

Thank yourself for your good work. (Pause)

If your eyes are closed, open them whenever you are ready.
Feeling fully alert, yet very relaxed.

Children's Mindfulness Meditation 5: Treasure Island – Discovering Inner Gifts

Ages: 5-12 ~ Meditation: 10-15min. ~ Activities: 30-45 min.

Warm-up, Meditation & Follow-up Activities

I. Warm-up

Introduction of Topic:

Please choose one of the following activities:

- To introduce the ocean theme, bring in a variety of seashells. Have children touch and explore. Talk about the different colors, shapes, and sizes. Talk about life and animals in the ocean.
- To introduce a nautical theme, bring in books about different kinds of ships and life aboard a ship. Discuss. Also, talk about the different parts of a ship (i.e. anchor, sails) and their importance.
- To introduce the concept of how each of us is special and unique, talk about what "Inner Gifts" are; talk about what the children like about themselves and what they think makes them special.

Opening questions:

To spike interest in the upcoming meditation, ask questions like:

- Have you ever had the opportunity to travel on a ship?
- What does it feel like to live aboard a ship?
- What are things you like about yourself? Name three.

Give children time to think and answer each question!

Fun Activities:

Please choose one of the following activities:

- Treasure Hunt: Hide small trinkets around the room beforehand. Have children hunt for "treasures".
- Scavenger Hunt with nautical or ocean theme, or "Discovering Inner Gifts" theme: Prepare different stations with instructions beforehand (i.e. "Find three seashells", "Draw a ship", "Name three things you like about yourself", etc.).

II. Mindfulness Meditation 5: Treasure Island – Discovering Inner Gifts

- Encourage (but don't force!) children to close or cover their eyes during the meditation.
- Have children choose their own meditation posture (i.e. sitting, laying, etc.). Let them choose a meditation position they feel most comfortable with.

24

- Turn to page 26 for the meditation script. Read thoughtfully; allow time for children to process what they are experiencing while you are reading.
- When you are done reading, give children time to slowly "wake up" and stretch. When all children are fully alert, continue with the Follow-up activities outlined below.

III. Follow-up Activities

Discussion Questions:

Discussing what children experienced during meditation can help with processing thoughts and feelings, thus deepening the effects.

Here are ideas for conversation topics:

- How are you feeling?
- What did you experience during the meditation (i.e. see, hear, feel)?
- How will you use what you experienced in this meditation in your daily life? Concretely, when, where, and how will you use it?
- Who would you want to take with you next time and why? Who else?

Please remember: there are no wrong answers. Simply thank children for contributing to the question or ask them to describe the experience further.

Creative Arts Projects:

Creative Arts Projects can deepen the effects and understanding of children's meditation. The following are ideas to do together.

Please choose one of the following activities:

- Draw, paint, or make a collage out of magazine clippings of a Treasure Island map. Where is your treasure hiding? What does your island look like?
- Draw or paint the ship called "Courage". What does a ship called "Courage" look like?
- Draw your animal friends from the Treasure Island Meditation: the parrot, dolphins, seabirds, etc.
- Draw your treasure chest.
- Draw what the golden mirror shows you. Draw what you saw in the mirror.
- Draw the crystals that reflect pictures of people and animals you love and cherish.
- Bake a Treasure Island cake and decorate it.
- Make a treasure chest out of heavy paper stock, construction paper, or cardboard. Decorate it.
- Draw, paint, or make a collage of the experiences or feelings you had during the meditation.
- Imaginary Play: Pretend-play the Treasure Island Story.
- Make sand art. Fill clear screw cap bottles with layers of different colored sand.

Encourage children to share their projects with the group!

Meditation Script 5: Treasure Island – Discovering Inner Gifts

Imagine you are the captain of a ship. (Pause)

Your ship's name is "Courage".
Its body is made out of wood called "Strength". (Pause)

You feel the gentle waves of the ocean peacefully rocking you up and down.
Your trusted companion, a wise parrot, is right by your side.
Together you have mastered many adventures.
If you ever need help or advice, your friend is there for you. (Pause)

A family of cheerful dolphins joins the voyage.
You hear the seabirds playfully singing their song.
They are your friends. (Pause)

When you look up above at the rich blue sky, you see puffy white clouds smiling at you. (Pause)

Notice how peaceful it feels. (Pause)

The air smells fresh and clean. (Pause)

Take a deep breath in.
As you breathe out, notice how refreshing the air feels. (Pause)

High up in the sky you see the North Star.
The North Star is the brightest star in the sky.
It is always visible, day and night.
It is there for you, to guide you wherever you would like to go. (Pause)

Today, the North Star is guiding you to a very special place called Treasure Island. (Pause)

When you arrive at Treasure Island, you release the big, sturdy anchor of your ship.
It gently and swiftly glides through the water:
down,
down,
down,
gently and swiftly,
further down,
past the corals and colorful fish,
past the rocks,
and all the way down to the ocean floor. (Pause)

TREASURE ISLAND - DISCOVERING INNER GIFTS

The anchor feels so strong and grounded as if it were connected to the center of the earth.
Feel how centered the anchor holds your ship. (Pause)

With the ship safely secured, you step off to explore the island. (Pause)

Close by, you see beautiful green palm trees swaying in the gentle breeze. (Pause)
The sand beneath your feet feels warm and soft. (Pause)

There, in a hidden cove, you notice something shiny glistening in the bright sunlight.
As you come closer you see a big, heavy treasure chest. It has shiny golden buckles and hinges.
Go ahead and open it.
You may hear a slight creaking sound as if the chest hasn't been opened for quite some time. (Pause)

What you find within the treasure chest might surprise you:
There are precious jewels containing your favorite memories.
You notice a golden cup that is overflowing with your favorite feelings.
Precious crystals reflect pictures of people and animals you love and cherish.
The treasure chest contains everything that makes you feel good about yourself and others. (Pause)

There is also a golden mirror.
When you pick up the mirror and look at it, you notice something special.
It shows you who you are on the inside:

You see a loving heart that is filled with love for all beings: people, animals, plants and, of course,
yourself. (Pause)

The mirror also shows you all the gifts and talents you have that make you special. (Pause)

Please know that you are loved just the way you are, fully and completely, always. (Pause)

Take a moment to notice how you feel. (Pause)

Know that you can always come back to this special place any time you wish. (Pause)

When you are ready, go back aboard your ship. Your friends, the dolphins and seabirds, are waiting
for you to bring you back home. (Pause)
Thank your friends and yourself for the wonderful experience you've just shared. (Pause)

If your eyes are closed, open them whenever you are ready.
Feeling fully alert, yet very relaxed.

Children's Mindfulness Meditation 6:
Magic Carpet Ride – Strengthening Inner Awareness

Ages: 5-12 ~ Meditation: 15-20 min. ~ Activities: 30-45 min.

Warm-up, Meditation & Follow-up Activities

I. Warm-up

Opening Questions:

To spike interest in the upcoming meditation, ask questions like:

- Have you ever wanted to travel on a Magic Carpet?
- What would it be like?
- How big would your Magic Carpet be?
- Would it have a pillow or chair? Or bed?
- Who would you want to take with you?
- What place or places would you go visit?
- How do you think it would look, feel, and sound there?

Give children time to think and answer each question!

Fun Activity:

- Have children sit on a colorful Play-Parachute representing the Magic Carpet. Pull them gently across the room. Create "waves". Have another adult or child help you turn the parachute in a circle. Change direction every once in a while.

II. Mindfulness Meditation 6: Magic Carpet Ride – Strengthening Inner Awareness

- Encourage (but don't force!) children to close or cover their eyes during the meditation.
- Have children choose their own meditation posture (i.e. sitting, laying, etc.). Let them choose a meditation position they feel most comfortable with.
- Turn to page 30 for the meditation script. Read thoughtfully; allow time for children to process what they are experiencing while you are reading.
- When you are done reading, give children time to slowly "wake up" and stretch. When all children are fully alert, continue with the Follow-up activities outlined below.

III. Follow-up Activities

Discussion Questions:

Discussing what children experienced during meditation can help with processing thoughts and feelings, and thus deepen the effects.

Here are ideas for conversation topics:

- How are you feeling?
- What did you experience during the meditation (i.e. see, hear, feel)?
- How will you use your experience from this meditation in your daily life? Concretely, when will you use it and how?

Additional questions you might ask:

- What did your Magic Carpet look like?
- How did you experience the ride on your Magic Carpet?
- What did you see, feel, or hear at the place you landed?
- Would you like to share the special message you received?
- Where would you like to go next?
- Can you remember a time where you wished you had your Magic Carpet?
- When do you think you may need the Magic Carpet again?

Please remember: there are no wrong answers. Simply thank children for contributing to the question or ask them to describe their experience further.

Creative Arts Activities:

Creative Arts Projects can deepen the effects and understanding of children's meditation. The following are ideas to do together.

Please choose one of the following activities:

- Draw your Magic Carpet or create a collage out of various materials.
- Make your own Magic Carpet. Use various art supplies such as fabric, yarn, fabric paint, etc.
- Draw or paint your Guide. What did you learn from your Guide?
- Draw or paint the place where the Magic Carpet took you. Draw what you saw, heard, and smelled.
- Draw or write down the special message you received. Roll up the note and put a colored ribbon around it. Put the note inside a special container, like a glass or tin jar. Help children find a special place for it.
- Create a book or journal with pictures, or write down what you experienced during the meditation.
- Draw or paint a picture of the experiences or feelings you had during the meditation.

Encourage children to share their project with the group!

Meditation Script 6: Magic Carpet Ride – Strengthening Inner Awareness

Imagine a warm summer evening.
You are walking in a beautiful meadow with luscious green grass and flowers in all the colors of the rainbow. (Pause)

The path beneath your feet feels soft.
Birds are singing in the trees. (Pause)

A steady breeze is gently rustling the leaves, playing a beautiful musical melody.
The air smells fresh and clean. (Pause)

You take a deep breath in.
And then release the air. (Pause)

Again, take a deep breath in.
Release the air. (Pause)

And one more time: deep breath in.
And release. (Pause)

Feel how relaxed you are. (Pause)

In the distance you notice an inviting campfire.
The warm glowing light of the campfire illuminates the rich blue sky. (Pause)

What is this? You wonder as you get closer. (Pause)

As you near the softly glowing campfire, you feel the warmth and light on your body. (Pause)

Focus the attention on your heart. Imagine there is a warm, golden light.
As you breathe into your heart, the warm, golden light fills you with love. (Pause)

Feel the love and light travel throughout your body. (Pause)

Feel the warm, loving glow as it flows slowly down your arms, softly spilling into your hands until finally spreading to the tip of each of your fingers. (Pause)

Now feel the light traveling down your body into your legs. Feel the warm, golden light reach your feet, and then travel to each toe. (Pause)

Now that you see and feel your body filled with light and warmth, also see your heart filled with love and light for all beings: people, animals, and plants. They all are your friends. (Pause)

Can you feel your heart grow bigger and warmer? It's getting bigger and warmer because of all the love you experience. (Pause)

By the golden glowing campfire, your Guide is waiting for you. Your Guide may be your Guardian Angel, an old wise being, an animal, or an imaginary being you feel you have known for a long time and you know you can trust. (Pause)

Everyone has their own Guide. That Guide takes care of you and protects you, always.
Your Guide is always with you, and you are never alone. (Pause)
Remember this, and know that you are loved.
Know that you always have someone who looks after you and cares for you with love. (Pause)

Your Guide warmly greets you and takes you to a clearing hidden behind a circle of bushes. (Pause)

There, between the tall grass and beautiful flowers, lies a Magic Carpet.

Notice the colors in your Magic Carpet.
What colors do you see? (Pause)

Put your hands on the Magic Carpet and feel its surface. What does the Magic Carpet feel like?
Does it have a rough surface? Or is it smooth? (Pause)

Your Guide invites you to take a ride on the Magic Carpet.
Before you step on the Magic Carpet, notice a Worry Box sitting on the ground next to it. (Pause)

Imagine putting your worries, and anything you want to let go of, inside that box.
The box will take all kinds of worries, be it with your friends, family, or school.
The Worry Box accepts anything you would like to put inside. (Pause)

The Magic Carpet is ready for you now.
Go ahead and sit down on it. (Pause)

Check within yourself: Do I have everything I need to feel safe and comfortable?
Or is there something I need?
If yes, ask your guide to get that for you. (Pause)

Notice how you feel. (Pause)

continued on page 32

When you are ready, get comfortable and prepare for takeoff. (Pause)

The Magic Carpet already knows where to take you.
This may be in the past, the present, or the future.
The Magic Carpet knows exactly where to go. (Pause)

As you take off, feel the breeze on your body. (Pause)

Your Guide is right beside you. Together, the two of you enjoy the view as the Magic Carpet gently glides through the air.
Relax and enjoy the ride. (Pause)

When the Magic Carpet lands, get ready to step off. (Pause)

Take a look around. What do you see?
Are you in nature?
Or are you in a city? Or a village? (Pause)

Listen for sounds.
What do you hear?
Do you hear birds?
The wind?
Or maybe you hear music? (Pause)

Notice any smells in the air that remind you of something or somebody. (Pause)

What does it feel like where you are? (Pause)

If there is something that interests you, go ahead and move closer. (Pause)

Remember your Guide is always with you and it is safe to explore. (Pause)

Are there any people around?
Imagine feeling comfortable enough to ask them where you are. (Pause)

You can also ask your Guide.
Listen for the answer. (Pause)

Take a moment to find out if there is anything you need to hear, see, or feel while you are here. (Pause)

Know that you can always come back to this special place and explore further. (Pause)

When you are ready, return to the Magic Carpet. (Pause)

Get comfortable and have the Magic Carpet take you home. (Pause)

Relax and enjoy the ride.
Thank yourself and your Guide for the experience you've just shared. (Pause)

When you arrive, park the Magic Carpet back in its hiding place at the clearing behind the circle of bushes.
Step off the Magic Carpet and return to the warm, softly glowing campfire. (Pause)

Notice how peaceful it feels. (Pause)

Perhaps your heart is filled with peace and gratitude as well. (Pause)

Send these feelings back to the Universe for the highest and greatest good. (Pause)

If your eyes are closed, open them whenever you are ready.
Feeling fully alert, yet very relaxed.

Children's Mindfulness Meditation 7: One Minute Peace – Quick Relaxation Practice

Ages: 6-12 ~ Meditation: 5-10 min. ~ Activities: 30-45 min.

Warm-up, Meditation & Follow-up Activities

I. Warm-up

Introduction of Topic:

Please choose one of the following activities:

- Bring in different symbols of peace (i.e. a picture of a dove, the universal peace sign, an olive branch, a white flag, or the peace hand symbol, etc.). Show and discuss with the children. Talk about what peace is.
- Read a short story or book about peace.
- Talk about Nobel Peace Prize Winners. What did they do? What did they stand for?
- Have you ever helped make peace happen? How did you feel?

Opening Questions:

To spike interest in the upcoming meditation, ask questions like:

- What does peacefulness feel like? Have children give examples of when and where they felt peaceful.
- How are peacefulness and relaxation connected?
- What is relaxation good for?

Give children time to think and answer each question!

Fun Activity:

- Draw or paint your own peace symbol.

II. Mindfulness Meditation 7: One Minute Peace – Quick Relaxation Practice

- Encourage (but don't force!) children to close or cover their eyes during the meditation.
- Have children choose their own meditation posture (i.e. sitting, laying, etc.). Let them choose a meditation position they feel most comfortable with.
- Turn to page 36 for the meditation script. Read thoughtfully; allow time for children to process what they are experiencing while you are reading.
- When you are done reading, give children time to slowly "wake up" and stretch. When all children are fully alert, continue with the Follow-up activities outlined below.

III. Follow-up Activities

Discussion Questions:

Discussing what children experienced during meditation can help with processing thoughts and feelings, thus deepening the effects.

Here are ideas for conversation topics:

- How are you feeling?
- What did you experience during the meditation (i.e. see, hear, feel)?
- How will you use what you experienced in this meditation in your daily life? Concretely, when, where, and how will you use it?

Please remember: there are no wrong answers. Simply thank children for contributing to the question or ask them to describe the experience further.

Creative Arts Projects:

Creative Arts Projects can deepen the effects and understanding of children's meditation. The following are ideas to do together.

Please choose one of the following activities:

- Draw or paint your heart filled with love and peace. You can also make a collage with magazine clippings.
- Draw or paint how breath travels through the body.
- Draw or paint a picture of the experiences or feelings you had during the meditation.
- Draw or paint three things in your life you feel peaceful about.
- Write a poem or draw a picture about what peacefulness means to you.

Encourage children to share their projects with the group!

Meditation Script 7: One Minute Peace – Quick Relaxation Practice

Gently close your eyes.
You can also put your hand over your eyes. (Pause)

Take a deep breath in.
Feel your tummy and chest rise. (Pause)

Slowly breathe out and let all the air leave your lungs. (Pause)

Again, take a deep breath in.
Feel your tummy and chest rise. (Pause)

Slowly breathe out and feel how the air leaves your lungs. (Pause)

One more time: breathe in.
Feel your tummy and chest rise. (Pause)

Slowly breathe out and relax your body. (Pause)

Keep focusing on your breath.
Breathe in and out. (Pause)

Every time you breathe in, feel your tummy and chest rise.
Every time you breathe out, feel your body relax further. (Pause)

Feel all the tension in your body release.
Notice the muscles in your arms and legs become smooth and soft. (Pause)

Listen to your breath.
Breathe in and out. (Pause)

Relax your mind.
Let go of all your worries and concerns.
See them drift away. (Pause)

Breathe in and out. (Pause)

Open your heart.
Let in peace and love. (Pause)

Allow yourself one minute of feeling at absolute peace.

(1min. Pause)

When you are ready, go ahead and open your eyes.
Feeling fully alert, yet very relaxed.

About the Author

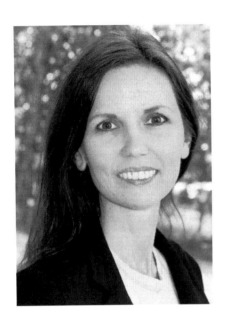

Dr. Nicola Kluge, Ph.D. specializes in helping children, parents and teachers succeed in school and at home.

She is a certified Creative Arts Therapist and Children's Mindfulness Instructor.

Originally from Germany, she lives with her husband and four children in Texas, USA.

Her hobbies include taking care of rescue dogs, reading, Yoga, and Photography.

Other Products

For Free Mindfulness Activities
Connect with Us at
MindfulnessForKids.net

Check out our "Mindfulness For Kids" series: books, CDs and MP3s.

If you enjoyed this book please leave a review online.
Thank you for your support!

27347576R00024

Made in the USA
Middletown, DE
16 December 2015